LOO[illegible]
LOOKI[illegible]G BACK –
Happy Memories, That's a Fact

by
Sharon Rose

Five years on, author of
Single Salsa Survivor:
The Journal of a Breast-Cancer Survivor

ARTHUR H. STOCKWELL LTD
Torrs Park, Ilfracombe, Devon, EX34 8BA
Established 1898
www.ahstockwell.co.uk

British Library Cataloguing-in-Publication Data.
A catalogue record for this book is available from the British Library.

By the same author:
Single Salsa Survivor
Living in Grief, Loving in Grief
Always Sublime, Never Ridiculous

Personal logo
By
Kathryn Robbins Artist
Carina Rixner graphic designer
Thank you
Sharon

ISBN 978-0-7223-4565-8
Printed in Great Britain by
Arthur H. Stockwell Ltd
Torrs Park Ilfracombe
Devon EX34 8BA

Dedication

Thank you, DAD, for being you, without you in the world there would have been no ME, but because of you I have experienced the joy of music and song. You left me a legacy, your eccentricity. At least in life we have always managed to laugh I say cheerio until we meet again.

"Wish me luck as you wave me goodbye."

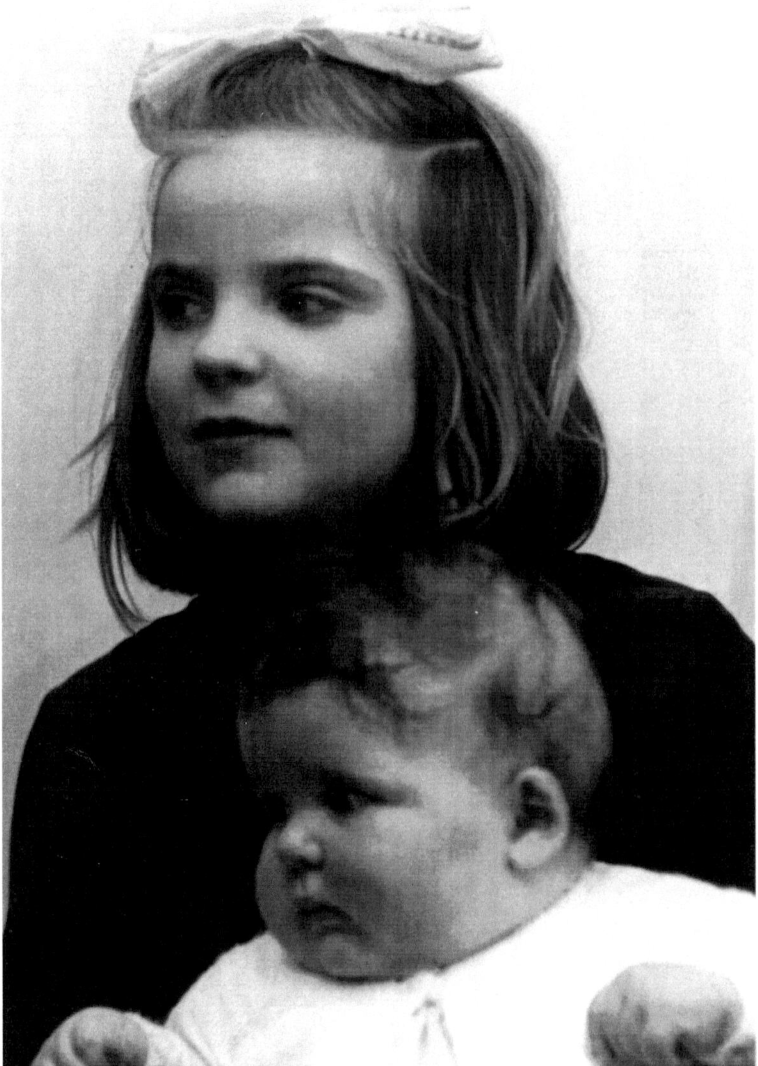

Author aged six and a half years old and her sister,
Helen aged six months.

Preface

From Adversity to Creativity

When I think back to my days as a student nurse in the 70s – sitting in my very small but cosy room in the nurses' home listening to my records, relaxing after a very exhausting but equally rewarding shift on the ward – I remember my desire to express my feelings through the written word and whilst my friends had pictures of Sting from the pop group The Police on their walls, I would have scraps of paper stuck on the wall with Sellotape, poetry I had written. It was all part of my inherited eccentricity and my friends thought I was good fun but maybe a little quirky. The poems at that time in my life were humorous *when life was carefree and fun!*

I finished my nurse training and started a lifelong career in the NHS: midwifery training, marriage and children followed. The creative part of my soul lay dormant and it wasn't until the age of forty-five years of age that I found that I had a passion and addiction for salsa dancing, but at the same time my life was to change dramatically for me and my family. I was diagnosed on one cold November day in 2005 with breast cancer. I didn't have the attention span to read much and so I kept a journal of how I felt through treatment for cancer and continued to record a diary of events into my remission. Before I knew it, my journal started a journey of its own.

In 2006 I had no spare money for Christmas presents and so with the help of a friend I typed my journal and gave it to my family, children and friends with a CD of my favourite songs that had touched my heart during those long and painful days during cancer treatment. I wanted them to know how much I appreciated their love and kindness through this most difficult time in my life.

The feedback I had from my family and friends about my journal was that I should try and get the story published because they did feel it may help other cancer sufferers and those who love them understand the effect cancer has on the person and all those that love and care for that person. I waited patiently to approach publishers with my manuscript because the book I wanted to publish was to be a positive book or none at all. I wanted to put on the bookshelf in the shops a story of survival, a story to reflect the exuberance of living and the ability to embrace uncertainty.

In March 2010 Arthur H. Stockwell Ltd published my book *Single Salsa Survivor: The Journal of a Breast-Cancer Survivor*, my second book, *Living in Grief, Loving in Grief*, was published in October 2011 and my third book, *Always Sublime, Never Ridiculous*, celebrates my five-year anniversary of surviving cancer. Donations from books sales are made to national and local cancer charities.

Cancer took away my mortality but gave me and

my family a new-found vitality in life. The power to share life experience through the written word. For the next nine years I have Raced for Life for CRUK and been a media volunteer, with TV and radio appearances, raising the profile of CRUK.

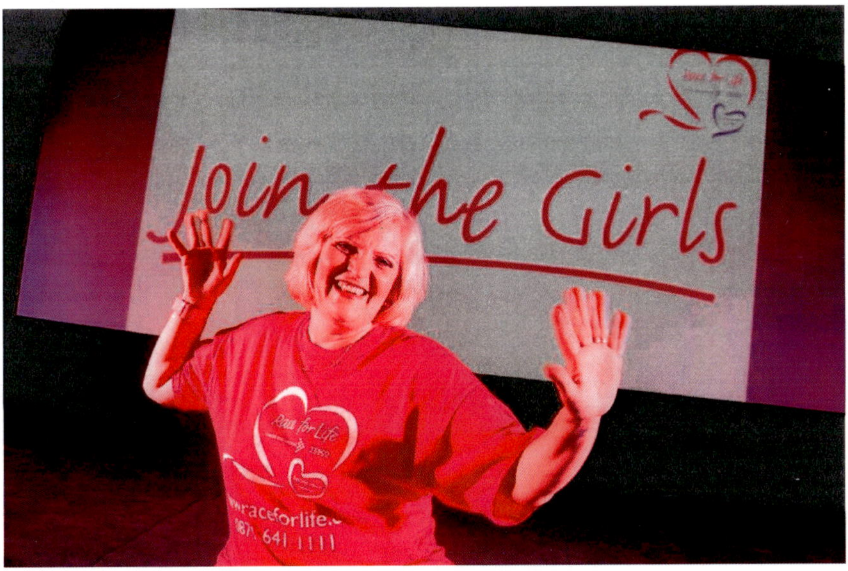

As a media volunteer.
Race For Life, 'The Musical' 2011.

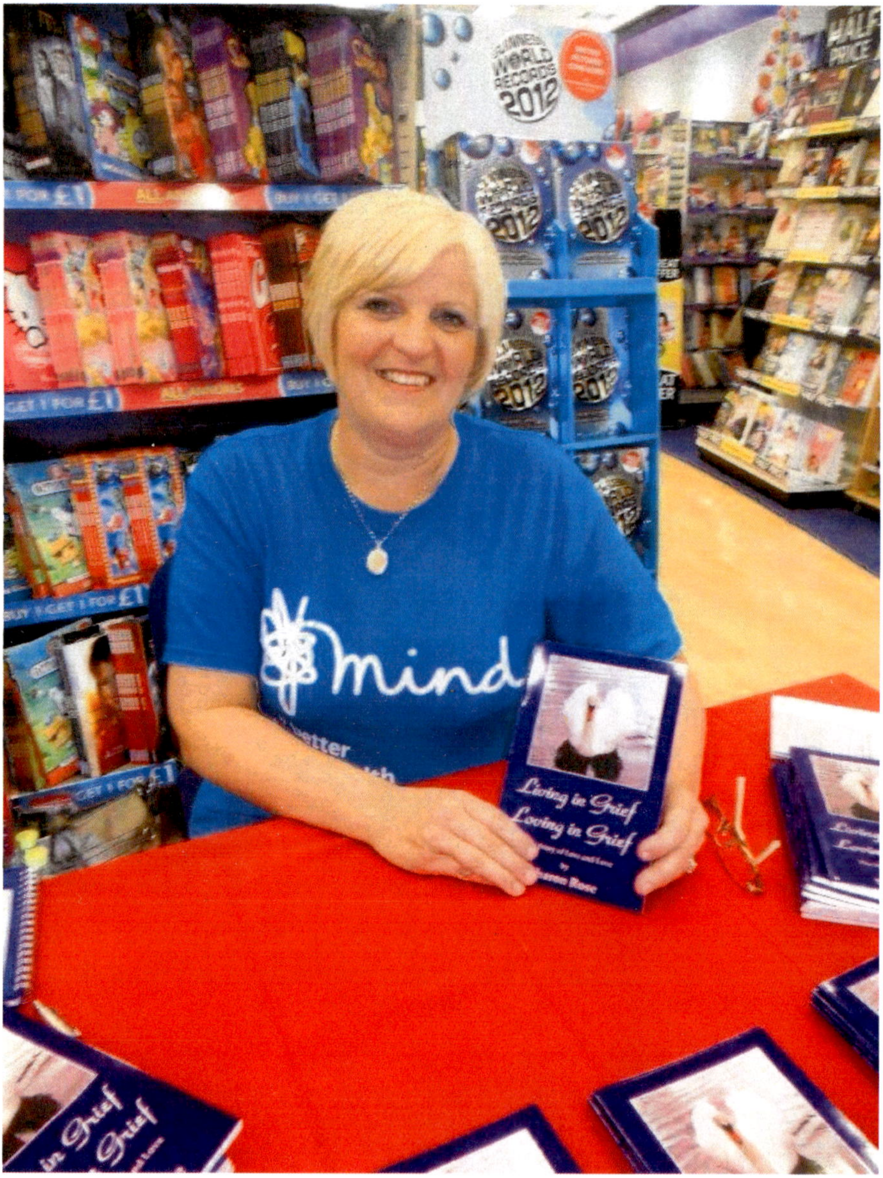

The author at WH Smith with her second book, 2012.
Supporting the Samaritans and Cruse Bereavement Care, Staffordshire.

Looking In, 14 February 2011

We exchange Valentine's cards of love, we are still newly-weds me and Chris, but newly-weds with baggage, in fact my suitcases are very heavy at the moment, I hold one handle and Chris is holding the other. With all that comes with caring for my chaotic firstborn daughter and being a mum and Chris a dad to a four-year-old granddaughter whose emotions are so fragile at the moment. Her dual heritage is now the topic of conversation in our household instigated by Erica, Erica wants to be the colour peach, and wants to have blonde hair. "Why am I Brown?" she asked me. I in desperation dyed my hair brown. I did seek advice because in the town where I live there is a very low ethnic minority. I visited a local Caribbean society to help her identify more with her colour, culture and identity. Then it dawned on me that Erica needed to feel good about herself, the magic words 'a healthy self-esteem' whatever her colour, culture, Erica had to feel beautiful inside and out. All settled down and then out of the blue I had a telephone call from her dad wanting to see her and the jigsaw was complete. Her contact with her culture and her heritage all seemed to make sense. The best thing to happen and now Erica has a dad, a stepmum and a brother, a family that love her.

The outside external pressures did put pressure on our new marital bliss and for one day and one day only Chris dropped the handle of the suitcase and ran away into his cave leaving me on my own, alone again. The load was heavy but not as heavy as my heart.

I could not blame him for leaving. I cried and felt very sorry for myself, but there was not much I could change. This story begins with the philosophy and debate about unconditional love. The love that ties me to my daughter's chaotic lifestyle and her erratic random impulsive personality controlled so much by a soul trapped in a self-indulgent world. The chemical imbalance in a chaotic brain can sometimes leave her open to exploitation from not very nice people. A world that breeds weakness, addiction, conflict and sadness, not at all what I envisaged for my daughter's future. I know one thing for certain, I didn't want it for me either, but with gritted teeth I sometimes had to enter her chaotic world to just for one moment hold her in my arms and protect her from not the outside world but herself. As the years go by my resolve for stress is weakening and life in general after cancer was leaving me as my friend Kathryn would say: "Keep calm we are pebbles!"

Looking Back

I didn't really notice until Fiona was about five that there was anything out of the ordinary or different about my daughter, and in fairness there have been many environmental factors that have contributed to the question of whether Fiona's chaotic lifestyle stems from childhood experiences or the label of possible Asperger's syndrome. A divorce, her mum remarrying, a new baby, moving to a new town, separation from her dad except for weekends, and so on. Therefore it was sometimes difficult to establish whether seeing her rocking on the settee or pulling her hair out, fidgeting and the tics that developed over the years were caused by emotional upheaval or something else that a diagnosis may have helped Fiona and her family understand her. Fiona had a special ability for remembering pop songs word for word and singing became her passion, she would spend hours singing in her bedroom to Disney's *Pocahontas* and *The Lion King*. For many years Fiona would enter singing and beauty competitions, recording her own songs in the studio. Just as her mum writes books, Fiona writes her own lyrics. We did have unpredictable moments with Fiona like the times she would run away up the road because she didn't like the smell of fruit gums. Fiona hated a change in routine, holidays were traumatic, Fiona didn't want to be cuddled and she would avert her gaze so as not to sustain eye contact with me. Asperger's was mentioned by the paediatrician but we carried on the best we could dealing with a little girl with a big eccentric personality. When she was good she was very very good and when she was bad she was 'orrid! Fiona had to deal with the fact she was a stepdaughter and as much as he tried her stepdad made it obvious that he found Fiona difficult to handle, probably because she was like her mum in lots of ways and after fifteen years of marriage I decided the rest of my life would be better spent with just my children and without them being exposed to any further conflict. My children came first and their health and well-being always will.

When Fiona was a child and young adult I had some parental power to protect her from herself but when she was eighteen I destroyed all the childhood letters from the paediatrician to give her a chance to enter adulthood without any evidence of a label. I thought it would be a fresh start. Fiona since the age of sixteen had fairly healthy relationships and I began to fall into a false sense of security and began to think everything was cured by that transition into adulthood. I had once been told that parenting is not ever finished until the day your child can live independently without you. Fiona's career choices were modelling and then pole dancing. Debate and discussion followed, but she enjoyed dancing and she was determined to fight society and stereotypical judgement. She stood her ground and claimed she was of course in the entertainment business.

Then came along our precious gift Erica, Fiona's daughter. I loved and cared for my daughter throughout her pregnancy and at the same time I was in the process of cancer treatment: chemotherapy and radiotherapy. A week after the treatment finished I jumped into my next role as birthing partner. I keep trying to cut those apron strings, but I just couldn't break free from strings coated in a lethal substance called unconditional love. I found it easy not to like my child sometimes but impossible not to love her.

Five years later in 2011 Fiona is pregnant again and that is another story, all I know is that I am to venture on a forty-week roller-coaster that will again challenge my physical and emotional stamina. Surviving cancer has set a benchmark for my tolerance and ability to cope and rise to a new challenge but that doesn't mean to say I am Superwoman at this moment.

I came home and expected a dark, cold place, but I had a surprise in store: the fire was burning and the living room was cosy and Chris sat on the sofa with a smile.

Chris picked up the other handle of the case and promised to carry the heavy load with me, in turn halving the worry and sometimes holding the case whilst I regained strength to carry on again. I embraced the fact his bubbling and positive persona filled the empty atmosphere again and I was glad.

So life was to carry on, as we thought, firefighting the chaos together.

Twenty-four hours later laughter again turned into tears.

Looking In

It was Wednesday 16 February 2011, slimming club night. Helen (my sister) and I had decided to go for it and try to lose weight and get fit. In previous weeks we had joined a fitness group on a Monday morning and there we laughed and laughed as we danced Bollywood, soon we were going to try a little Zumba. I had lost 7 lb in weight and was really pleased with the results; Helen had not lost weight and I said to her, “I am not coming with you again if you keep eating those Penguin biscuits.” At the same time each week I had noticed that she had started to look very pale. I had no way seen her this pale before, I had told her I was worried about her but she reassured me about a recent scan, and that everything was fine. Uhmmm, but was it? I was focusing on the healthy diet, I had made space in my mind and life to concentrate on myself for a change. My appointment for my five-year mammogram and health check was looming and I was very nervous of what this was to entail, most of all the results. I had learnt to cope in between appointments and get on with life, after five years of life after cancer I had even started whining about the trivia, but I was not quite as bad as in precancerous times. What I was enjoying at the moment was quality time with my sister. We had very different personas but a strong sisterly bond. We were never far away from each other especially in times of hardship. Helen had always been there for me in the last few years through chemotherapy, supported me with Erica and looked after Erica while I had a week’s break with Chris holidaying in the Canaries. If I could win the lottery I would pay for my sister and her family to enjoy the holiday of a lifetime, but knowing my sister she would choose a summer at our mum and stepdad Mike’s caravan with her family and the new addition Rose Button, the family Dalmatian puppy.

With a similar outlook on life although different in personality we sisters were bought up by the same strong woman to have family values and loyalties, we never argued and we respected each other's views, we were open and honest and loved each other, complemented each other's strengths whilst respecting each other's weaknesses. My quietly confident caring sister became my strength when we lost our brother when he took his own life. Her renewal of her Catholic faith and her calm, collected manner supported me through our loss. I am a heart-on-the-sleeve, on-the-edge person. I don't think I would have been able to handle my brother's death without her.

Helen wants to talk to me before we venture into the world of pro points. I was not prepared for what was to happen next. Our lives were to catapult us both on to that planet I visited not that long ago: Cancer Planet.

In a daze I am listening to what Helen has to say. "I have been to the hospital today," she said. "I need a partial nephrectomy. I have an 80% chance that a tumour found on the scan of my kidney is cancer."

What did you say? I think I misheard. I thought you said you have been diagnosed with possible renal cancer. Is this really happening or am I dreaming?

That evening we both had put on a pound, but I was quick to get out of the slimming club. I needed to go somewhere we could talk. That was the last time we went to the slimming club, losing weight fell into insignificance as we were both thrown into staying alive.

Cancer, the C word, that is my word *cancer*, it can only belong to me, I have managed that illness myself but all the family have lived on a knife-edge praying the cancer will not come back, living with uncertainty for five years. Three more weeks until my five-year check-up and mammogram and not just myself but all the people who love me might have had some freedom, a reason to celebrate and peace of mind. There is no guarantee attached to the check-up that all is going to be OK. I had already celebrated five years' survival in November 2010 in Gran Canaria on my honeymoon. The family will need to rewind right back to the beginning again, survival countdown. This cannot be happening! This family has had more than enough to contend with in the last few years. You cannot have said *cancer*. No, no, that is not in my life's plan.

You are the living memory of Adrian and myself, you're the one at the Bailey helm, you were the only person in the world I could leave this world in peace, knowing you would care for Erica as if she were your own. As we drink our latte I see in your face that this nightmare is real. I see it deep within your eyes, a steel glaze, the protection barrier is up and although you are looking back at me the soul has wrapped itself within a body now in fight-or-flight mode ready to take on the biggest challenge life can throw at you – SURVIVAL.

Let me in your mind
So I can read
Your every thought.
Let me share your pain
And protect you.
Please let me in.

I don't have to imagine
The pain you must feel.
I have been there
On cancer planet
Life is so surreal.

If you cry on my shoulder
I will console you.
If you laugh
I will laugh too.
If you want peace and quiet
To be by yourself
I will leave.
I am guided by you.

Please take my advice
Dwell only a while
On the sad, and the bad and the why.
Every second will count
So fight for your life.
You have every reason
Remember
So did I.

Looking Back, 21 January 2006

I remember, Helen, you taking me to my first ever appointment to see my oncologist and how I ran out of the building because I didn't want to walk through the doors with the sign that said 'Oncology' above the door. And the posters on the wall were about supporting people with cancer.

"I AM A NURSE,
GET ME OUTTA HERE!"

In January 2006 I walked through the doors on to the oncology ward in the Cancer Unit at the local hospital. I was very nervous and wanted to turn around and walk right back in time maybe just a month to when I was Health Visitor Service Manager. I walked on to the ward in anticipation. What new nursing skill was I going to learn today? What was I to learn about caring for the cancer patient?

My first observation was the diversity of the chemo population. Today, Treatment day for women with breast cancer, the ward was full – yes *full* – of ladies of varying ages and at different stages of treatment. Some of the ladies were quietly sitting talking to their relatives. It was difficult to distinguish who was the patient until you looked more closely at the hairline and saw a very neat, well-kept hairdo and realised it could be a wig. They were talking amongst themselves and the volunteers were busy making tea for both patient and relative and giving people hope of recovery as they told their own tales of surviving breast cancer years ago, and the patients and relatives bustled in the waiting area with protective comradeship for each other gaining strength from the fact they were all in the same boat.

Some women sat with all the same hairstyle, a black stubbly growth of hair just growing back and also a sign that they had come a long way they seemed to be able to relax more than the newcomers as if they felt a little more confident that they had got this far, and relieved they had managed to get halfway through their gruelling treatment. They were pale and dark under the eyes but there was an air of confidence, the ability to sit still for a few minutes and read magazines, instead of the newly diagnosed patient living on adrenalin and fear unable to read even a leaflet.

Then I ventured a little further down the ward to introduce myself to the nursing staff and I saw faces that told me the story of the cancer patient. The face in its most natural form, smooth transparent skin with no colour only pallor signifying such fragility, no eyebrows and no eyelashes and eyes so deep and meaningful there was no need for words. The eyes were the key.

The nurse has in her head knowledge at the ready to implement a programme of care to every individual patient. Care that has been well researched and documented as effective. The guidance from our hidden heroes the research scientists who tirelessly spend days and days in laboratories staring into microscopes to determine how we can cure this disease that takes lives indiscriminately. I have respect and still promote the importance of nursing education and training to the highest standard, recognising that nurses never become complacent and continue to remain accountable, updating their knowledge and skills to ensure the highest standard of nursing care.

To complement that necessary knowledge is to genuinely care about people.

The eyes hold the key to how your patient feels, how they are dealing with the physical or emotional pain, and how they are coping with their fear. Look into their eyes and you will see their most innermost, deepest emotions. When you look back at your patient make sure you convey in that second that you are listening to what they are saying, do not avert your gaze at the same time respecting territorial space and sometimes we prefer the phrase showing empathy rather than showing sympathy. The skill to care has to be there in your heart. These are essential criteria of any nurse's job description.

I sit down now and look into the eyes of the oncology staff nurse, and as I stare into her eyes I see a face so pale, I see fear, sadness. I look again and realise that in her eyes is a reflection. The reflection is MINE. Sure enough she looks back at me and touches my arm and just asks me, "How are you today?" and then she sits there administering my chemotherapy and listens to my stories not averting her gaze and she listens.

I relaxed and chatted away about all my fears and how I didn't want to leave my children, how I worried about my limited parenting ability and supporting my beautiful children emotionally through this traumatic time for them. It made me think of my role as a health visitor and the impact cancer has on all the family. My thoughts went to those young women undergoing treatment for cancer and trying to parent active young children. I walked out of the ward happy and reassured that I had been given the right treatment, by the right trained person with the right qualifications and most of all I so appreciated her kindness to me.

Thank you.

Chemotherapy finished and fifteen doses of radiotherapy later the only F word in my vocabulary was *fatigue* coupled with E for *elation* that I was alive. My short- and long-term goals just merged into one to stay **ALIVE**.

I prepared to return to work. I know some people work through their chemotherapy and that again is personal choice and very much job-dependent, but at the time of my diagnosis I was actually Health Visitor Service Manager and had been told that I would be returning to the front line due to NHS reorganisation. My manager at the time was a woman who had been locality manager for the NHS Trust for as long as I remember and I had great respect for her no-nonsense straight-talking but fair approach.

She called me into her office and said, "Sharon, you are going to be very vulnerable to infection, working with children is not the place to be whilst having chemotherapy. The time has come in your life and career to nurture yourself, to give yourself the best chance of recovery, now go home and begin self-preservation. I thank her to this day for showing me what a good manager should be. Thank you for being a caring manager. It meant a lot to me.

The lessons I learnt from a management perspective were to ensure full appreciation of a phased return to practice after such a serious illness.

To support that person back into the workplace I would suggest a very robust occupational health department involvement and utilise the counselling service.

Fatigue, fatigue – how much can I emphasise fatigue? Respect the fact that fatigue requires a phased return, and a good HR to look at the financial side of things will relieve some of the stress and worry. Then we have our own responsibility and accountability as regards our fitness to practice. We can seek help from our managers and unions for appropriate advice. There are also charities that support nurses who are going through difficult times, e.g. Cavell Nurses' Trust, not forgetting accessing help from national charities such as Cancer Research UK, Macmillan Cancer Support and of course talk to your breast care nurse specialist.

When the balance is right pick up your self-esteem and return to what you do best: your nursing career.

Looking In: Helen's Journey

On 5 March 2011 it was the second anniversary of our brother's death – well, when he was found by police as they battered down the barricade he had built behind his front door. His demise from this world was on 25 February 2009 when he took his own life and left us. Of all the dates in the year Helen had no choice but to have major surgery removing part of her kidney and taking out that dreaded tumour on the 5/3/2011.

The journey began two weeks ago, that is all, and

I know this roller-coaster ride, but I am a spectator and I see Helen twisting and turning up and down on this ride. I am helpless to reach her until she occasionally gets off and I hold her in my heart until she buys another ticket and again takes off on that roller coaster of life. It's a single ticket but it's not one way. No, it's solitary confinement for the duration of the ride then you get off the ride to come home to your family and some normality.

It's very different not being in control of your own illness, and I quiver helplessly unable to do a thing to take this away. I can help heal your wound, but only you can heal your mind.

From my perspective emotions are fragile. I have not experienced this before. Our brother threw us straight into grief. We had no choice, no influence on his life or his death.

I want to see you, my sister, every day to study your face and expressions to make sure you are not in pain. I can't believe it and therefore I keep asking you questions and you repeat the story about the finding of a tumour on your kidney. My mind has now only you in it. How can I help you, practically and emotionally, OMG how difficult can it be to know what to say, what to feel, when someone you love has cancer?

You want to do and say the right thing to make things OK, but I don't know how, do I?

I want to protect Helen from anything that will make her feel sad, unhappy, frightened, but I CANNOT protect her from life and the challenges cancer brings to her.

I want her to reassure ME, so I can handle it, I am worried in case you fall and reality kicks in, and I might not be there to catch you.

But then it's not about **ME**, is it?

I still have a part to play as your sister who loves you the best in the world and so my journey begins too. I see me squashed in a sidecar of a motorbike. I have to laugh at that image that comes to mind when I remember Olive out of *On the Buses*, for anyone who can remember the comedy of the 70s a comedy that made me laugh many years ago. I suppose there is some truth in the fact that as sisters we can always smile or laugh about something serious. No one else could possibly see the funny side, so I am sitting here in this sidecar shaking about seeing hazards ahead, trying to put the brakes on when I see a nasty bend in life and all I can do is shout and scream directions because you have the controls in your hands. I could grab the steering wheel if I wanted to but that is a big risk. Is it helping or interfering?

This leads me to the scenario when you wouldn't talk about your diagnosis and I couldn't see in your face what you were thinking, a closed door to the outside world. I was growing so frustrated because you hadn't discussed anything with your consultant, I had so many questions to ask – oh yes *I* again.

But in fairness it was only protection for you and you were getting stronger, strong enough to go into the outside world and meet people again. I had watched in awe as friends visited and spoke openly about the cancer and asked questions directly and you weren't phased. Why can't I ask you? Maybe it's the dynamics between friends and the difference between friends and family. Friends are totally focused on being helpful and confident in how they want to help. I am floundering in sisterly emotion and also don't ask because if I hear your inner thoughts could I bear the pain? You know that, and I know that as I go back years to my treatment. I would always put on a brave face for my family and shrug it off to protect their feelings. Ali, my son, once in an argument about their lack of understanding about how I felt, quite rightly pointed out that they only see me coping, strong, always smiling, blasé in fact, and Ali said I looked much worse at the end of my failing marriage.

That did teach me a valuable lesson about finding the balance in parenting about protecting children and keeping them from the nasty outside world and of course reality and the real parenting quality of supporting them with strategies to cope with what horrible curved balls life might throw at them.

How frustrated my close friends and family must have been and for just one moment I needed them to see I did understand the seriousness of my illness and that I was coping with it in my own way. I was frightened when I felt so ill as I had no alternative but to let my body take over my mind and lying there in my bed wonder if I was going to fade away to that unknown destination heaven at least; hell hadn't crossed my mind. So once I had an ounce of energy I was off that bed and permanently on a high, staying alive.

Helen, you visited our wonderful doctor, the most professional family GP. We were lucky to have someone with such expertise and kindness. You did finally get it in writing, you said only when you saw it in writing would you be able to comprehend and begin to know how to cope with your illness. So now you know, but you are such a private person, how you are handling the news is still very private.

I go to bed thinking about you and wake up thinking about you. What is the definition of that fear that grips my soul? I know it well and I have felt this fear before. I remember now it is the feeling of uncertainty. In *Single Salsa Survivor*, my first book published, I finally concluded that I had managed to embrace that uncertainty. I am thrown right back again to that feeling, a brief reminder but intense.

Weeks have passed and you have healed on the outside and inside you are living with the fact cancer touched you as we hope for just a short time.

How do I know you have been touched? Because you have a calmness about you, the calmness that characterises only those people who have been on Cancer Planet as I have. I have the luxury now of having something so precious in common with my sister and not the dreaded C word but the mutual love of such simple things like when we walk Rose Button in the fresh air, the trees look taller, the sun shines brighter, the grass is greener and the lake reflects our happiness to be here breathing in the breath of life. Beauty is not the expensive gifts or the colour of lots of money; beauty is me and you strolling by the lakes at the back of your house with your new addition to the family: Rose Button, a Dalmatian puppy.

There is not a book to write about Helen's journey because the pages belong to Helen. This chapter is about me and how I coped with the fact somebody I loved was diagnosed with cancer, and my message to relatives and friends is to keep it simple.

Be there
Be near
Be ready
To catch a tear.

The recent daily visits to the hospital to visit and care for my sister had taken me back in my career, in fact thirty years to the days when I was a young keen nurse thriving on adrenalin and love for my job. Whilst I was there at the hospital with Helen I met a nurse colleague from my training hospital in Birmingham. We hugged and reminisced about memories back in the day. Then I bumped into an old flame from my student nurse days. He's a consultant now and he hasn't changed a bit with his cheeky face and most endearing personality. I am glad he has done well in his career, he deserves it. He was a really sweet medical student with a lovely manner and lifted everybody's mood on the wards with his sense of humour. I am so glad that all those years ago as a student nurse I took my own Hippocratic oath not to sleep with doctors and thirty years later that oath has saved my ageing fifty-year face from embarrassment, plus the fact he married my friend.

That doesn't mean I didn't sleep with policemen or firemen, just not doctors. These encounters took me back in thought to such happy memories and reminded me how that young girl Sharon Bailey carved her career and how proud I am to this day to have worked in the NHS and I have enjoyed every single working day of my working life.

Looking Back, 1973

I had a vision of certainty in 1973. I was thirteen years of age and I knew from that day I wanted to be a nurse and midwife, my career set in stone. The only hurdle was the theoretical brain freezes that were to haunt me from GCSE to the age of thirty-one at university. Every – I mean *every* – examination I took I failed first time except my driving test. But then came resilience to overcome failure and the ability to try and try again. The power vocabulary is never using the sentence "I *Cannot* do it" but sometime we might assert ourselves and say, "I *Will Not* do it." The simple change in a sentence can make a difference to our self-confidence and self-esteem. The magic word is *choice*. Choices are there for most of our lives, it is only illness or worse death that can take away our choices.

My secondary school life was a mixed bag of pleasure and pain and I remember crying uncontrollably at a school disco to 'Ben' by Michael Jackson. I wasn't crying for the rat he was singing about, I was crying for myself and the collapse of my family life. Dad was sectioned under the Mental Health Act and had been institutionalised in the psychiatric hospital. He was never to come home again and living with schizophrenia for him and us didn't end until 18 June 2011 when Dad died at the age of eighty-one.

I was not alone and I would never ever be alone from the age of eleven to this present day because I had the definition of a reality BESTEST FRIEND, Janine, Joan, Gordon and her younger brother, Adrian. Ironically we have both lost our precious brothers.

The Tuesday after my best friend's wedding I

visited my second family after a day shift at the hospital. I had caught the bus and Joan and Gordon and Adrian and myself were all laughing as I gave them a rendition of my hymns I had chosen for my wedding. I loved Adrian as I did my own brother and he offered to drive me home in his very posh white sports Lamborghini. That was the last time I saw him. By Thursday evening he was dead, twenty-one years old killed in a car crash. How did I know? Because I received an urgent call whilst on duty on Friday morning to say on the ward down the hospital corridor were Adrian's friends injured from a car crash. I rushed to see them but the one face I wanted to see was not there. Adrian, my best friend's brother, lay in the mortuary. I was in charge of my own ward that day and I had to hold it together to see through the shift holding back a lifetime of tears and the desperate need to get to Joan and Gordon and share their grief. There was one further problem: Janine and Ian were on their honeymoon. They had to be contacted and post-wedding celebrations became funeral preparations. I grieved for a very long time and I remember even on my own honeymoon in Yugoslavia thinking that I kept seeing Adrian. I just couldn't bear the thought of not seeing him again.

The start of a lifetime of so many ups, downs, tragedies and joyous occasions – we have been through them all together. At eighteen we were in a nightclub on one of our traditional Thursday nights out and Janine met her soulmate Ian and for a lifetime we have been the Three Team. They are my soulmates and I am 'rock mother' to all their three girls and very proud to be part of their family. Janine and I only had a short time apart. Janine went to France to work at the age of sixteen/seventeen and I stayed on in the sixth form to retake all my GCSEs and set to attending interviews for a student nurse placement.

I managed to get the place, but had about six months before the course date, and there was no way I was going to spend that time doing nothing. Mum had given us the work ethos if you want something you have to work for it – and so my first ever interview was aged seventeen at a large impressive insurance company in Birmingham. A few months later, in the year 1977, I was called into the office, and my boss was eagerly waiting to tell me the company would like to finance my training to be an accountant. Oh dear me, now I was in a pickle. I was working here until May 1978 when I would start my nurse training. Choices to make and options to consider: a well-paid respectable profession and career in accountancy or my poorly paid dream as a nurse. I took the latter but I will always be grateful and honoured that the company thought I had potential to be an accountant considering I always struggled at mathematics. I was also an absolute menace in the office. I played terrible practical jokes on my colleagues. Iris, a mother-figure colleague, made me wear a ruler down the back of my clothes to try and correct my round shoulders. I made long-term friends who I nicknamed Bobbles and Debbles. Debbles was my friend and accomplice in the hilarity in the office. We decided to work overtime putting leaflets together in the printing department in the basement. Both of us had our ulterior motives. I was in love with the printing manager, who was married and much older than me, so I was happy to look and not touch. And that philosophy has always stayed with me all my romantic single life, married attached men OUT OF BOUNDS.

I never touch what is not mine to touch. But it passed the time and monotony of the job drooling over him. My friend's crush on Bobbles, who also worked in the printing department, was more fruitful. They fell in love and married with their favourite matchmaker (me of course) in tow as bridesmaid.

I have a reputation for going by the book and my upbringing was based on loyalty and honesty. I met with my boss and told him about my plans to be a student nurse and said I was actually going to hand my notice in in the very near future but thanked him for offering me such a great opportunity. He smiled and wished me luck and months later I cried as I left my first ever job and my first ever experience of the friendships formed in the workplace.

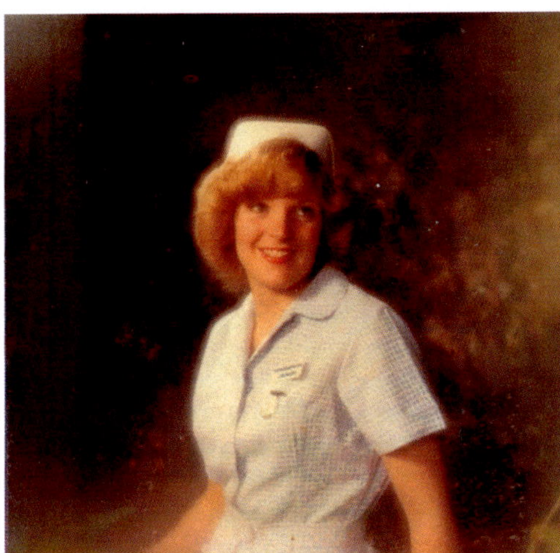

New Beginnings, 1978

I moved into the nursing home in May 1978, I left home and family and that was the start of a lifetime of happy memories as an adult who had flown the nest. This part of my life was to remain for ever consistent with my thirst to learn more and more about my profession, and what a journey that has been.

The anticipation is that every day you walk into work as a nurse you will not know what the day might bring and not one day until you retire will you ever in your career think you know everything. When you do retire there will be memories of people you met, those who lived those who died. The luxury of stepping into the world of people from all over the world, into their cultures. There is one rule to follow, the NMC code of conduct, plus academic research-based evidence, and finally the biggest topping of genuine concern and empathy for your fellow human beings.

A Hospital in Birmingham, UK, 1981

I am standing at the top of the ward, I am in charge of the ward today, a newly qualified staff nurse standing there proudly in my navy-blue dress and silver buckle and starched frilly white hat.

We were not allowed to wear uniforms outside of the hospital because of cross-infection. I had scurried across the path from the nursing home to the hospital, tightly wrapping my navy and red cape around my shoulders. I was unsure whether it was the cold winter morning air or the excitement of my first day as a staff nurse that made me shiver uncontrollably as I made my way to the medical ward.

I had just left the office after handover from the night. No computers in those days just the famous

Kardex, a flip notebook containing patients' every detail handwritten by nurses, a legal responsibility that still applies now. Notes on any patient contact have to be written within twenty-four hours in black ink.

For a very important moment of the day I stood still. I would capture every patient on the ward at that moment in my head as a benchmark of how they were feeling at the start of each new day ahead. It might be the only moment in the day when I would stay still in one place and then I would be off on my medicine round, on my feet all day and making important decisions on the go, delegating tasks to other nurse colleagues, supervising student nurses, highlighting at all times work within their scope of practice and encouraging them to feel comfortable to ask me anything that would increase their knowledge and skills to lead them to where I stand today, a competent trained nurse with the insight that today like any other day I will continue to learn something new. Nurses should have a degree in multitasking, it was an enormous responsibility to be responsible and ACCOUNTABLE for around thirty-three human beings who were actually dependent on your decisions for their lives.

I stood and looked carefully at every individual patient's face. I could detect the slightest change in their medical condition by just studying a facial expression. The colour of their skin, was it pale and wan? Were they in pain? Was their condition deteriorating? Or on the other hand was their face flushed because they were well and excited about the prospect of going home? Did they have a temperature? Were they brewing an infection?

Some wriggled in the bed. Were they in pain? Did they need help with repositioning in bed? Let's go and see, it may be as simple as plumping up the pillows, a bed pan, or commode, but let's just find out if they are OK. It's that simple.

Some had got back to bed and were sleeping peacefully, self-healing, pain-free and comfortable.

I could hear laboured heavy breathing and tuned in to every breath taken, these were my critically ill patients at the top of the ward near the office, for the obvious reason that we could see them. These patients required TLC – an abbreviation for tender loving care.

I am sure patients got to know this hierarchy on the ward and the happy faces sharing a joke or two down the bottom of the ward were those waiting to go home. After taking in quickly every individual I could assess priority workload for the nurses and delegate work appropriately.

Nurses were seen to be task-led in the day with two-hourly turns (pressure area care) to prevent pressure sores, sputum pot collection (yuk, you might say) and enemas for the most constipated. And the nurses smiled and listened intently on the doctors' rounds to the consultant who may have had the most verbal diarrhoea. It was my job to interpret the medical jargon to ensure the patient knew exactly what was going to happen to them next. I also made sure I knew every one of my patients and was able to recite their past twenty-four hours' hospital experience to the consultant on his rounds. Four-hourly observations of blood pressure, pulse, temperature recording, fluid input and of course measuring urine output meant we could build a picture of how the individual person was in the physical sense. Every pulse rate and temperature chart told a story and as I stood at the top of the ward and looked down at all my patients I collectively could see who needed my attention first. I could pre-empt a deterioration in a patient's condition. Single rooms of today I think hinder this even though they give privacy. Nurses today have to rely on the buzzer and there may be many wasted minutes before a patient will buzz the buzzer.

The making of beds with hospital corners, the rubbing of cream into ankles and elbows and of course bottoms, the emptying of bedpans all gave us the opportunity to have contact with our patient and make an assessment of their condition at every contact. This sounds for most people monotonous and task-orientated but it wasn't that bad. For nurses it's all in a day's work and an opportunity to pass the time of day with your patient. This could be a simple squeeze of the hand of the unconscious patient, a laugh and a bit of banter with the well and mobile, a time for tears and nurses to give a listening ear. A time to assess your patient's physical and emotional well-being.

When the long shift was nearing the end – it could be an early shift, or late shift, or night shift – I would be ready to crawl back to my tiny, tiny sanctuary of a room in the nurses' home. I would telephone Mum from a payphone in the corridor. If it was an early shift I might pop over for half a lager and blackcurrant at the hospital's local pub, then call in for chicken, chips and curry sauce – sorry, not very healthy but hey nurses are human too and not perfect but then that is what makes us human. I would wander home to my small cosy room in the nurses' home, play records on my old-fashioned stereo player and listen to the dulcet tones of soul singers Marvin Gaye and Al Green. On my wall was a display of my recent poetry. Little did I know I would become an author at the age of fifty. When I was a student nurse I had three years of working hard and all I remember is that it was a time in my life when I was so happy and fulfilled as a person.

Happy memories, that's a fact.

The hospital romances have always created intrigue and oh yes I had my doctor/nurse and dentist/nurse relationships. At one stage the medical students claimed I was the Marilyn Monroe of the hospital. Well, I felt like a movie star after that. The medical students were fun and quite cute in their white coats. But when the coffee break was over flirtations were over as soon as we stepped back on to the ward it was full concentration and not a step out of place that would compromise your patients' safety or medical care. I had a couple of altercations with psychiatrists but psychiatry touched a nerve with me, a nerve raw from the past.

Psychiatry was another experience in the 70s, institutions were still full of patients with long-term chronic mental illness. We worked twelve-hour shifts in psychiatry and conversations for those twelve hours never made much sense. It was wise not to challenge the patients as their behaviour was unpredictable. I think I felt the saddest because the disease of the mind is hard to cure. We would then take them on trolleys for their weekly ECT treatment. I searched for the reward in psychiatry and admired the nurses who dedicated their working life to just really making their lives just that little bit more bearable in their cruel world of schizophrenia, manic depression, personality disorder and so on. One of those patients used to walk around the hospital grounds. I could see him from my window but he couldn't see me – I didn't want him to see me. I was working on a ward that overlooked the grounds, and the man walked fast as if he had somewhere to go, important business to attend to but frustrated by the fact he was getting nowhere fast he stared at the ground. You could still see the strained features and agitation as he fought with demons telling him what to do. Those demons were not visible but clearly this man was agitated by them. I then saw nurses approaching him, their body language indicating they were using skills of negotiation to encourage the man to return to the ward taking care not to aggravate the situation, the nurses kept a little distance to protect themselves due to the unpredictability of the man. He could become violent. I looked again and a nurse had persuaded him to go with him back to his ward. I watched the man through the window, he was walking briskly still agitated.

His profile is very familiar, I know that man so well. I hold back a tear a tear of regret of sorrow of pity. Is the tear for the troubled broken man before my eyes or are the tears for the young nurse staring out of the window watching helplessly at the scene before her?

The nurse is me.

The man in the grounds I see from the window is my father.

Dad

I don't know what stage of grief I was at when I was eighteen and working in the very institution where my father was a patient. I think I had been through the grief process with my mother from the age of nine when the sweet, kind, funny man suddenly changed into a frightening ogre who tormented my mother, who smashed windows and doors. I would hide with my sister and brother behind the settee or hide in the downstairs lobby as we called the cloakroom, and with me was my frightened six-year-old sister and little toddler of a brother. For those early years I can only remember Mum crying with frustration, not knowing why this man she had loved and married and still loved questioned her faithfulness and marched her to the Catholic church to swear on the Bible that she had been faithful to him. I remember the smell of a man that lay in the bed for days not washing only sleeping, and I stared at this person from the bedroom door and there was a confused little girl who felt very guilty for hating her own father.

I really do not remember the exact date when my father's clever guise fell and the doctors eventually believed my own mum when she said the man she had married had died of a terrible illness that had took his heart, his soul and destroyed his mind and he was sectioned and institutionalised and I was glad, I was relieved. I was sad and guilty but peace and tranquillity once more became HOME.

In the 70s the treatment for the chaotic mind and chemical imbalance of the brain was electric-shock treatment and drugs to numb the thoughts that tortured the brain riddled with paranoia, and with a diagnosis of schizophrenia, my father lived quite happily in his own world and we as a family would visit him. I would at the age of thirteen catch two buses to visit him because our mum had taught us one value in life, loyalty.

Institutions were still large old buildings not a man's castle, but what seemed like an extension of a prison wall and this was the same for my father. A prison was right next door to the institution and the patients' lives were similar to those of the prisoners next door. This became a debate in the 70s and eventually care in the community decided to integrate patients with chronic mental health problems back into the community. I do not know what I think about that. Dad had his freedom back and he survived when he walked through the Birmingham riots, he had no fear at all but he was also vulnerable. He managed to get a credit card even though he had not worked for many years and purchased keyboards that became his only furniture in his inner-city flat. He would sit in his flat in the middle of his keyboard kingdom and just play happily for hours and hours his music.

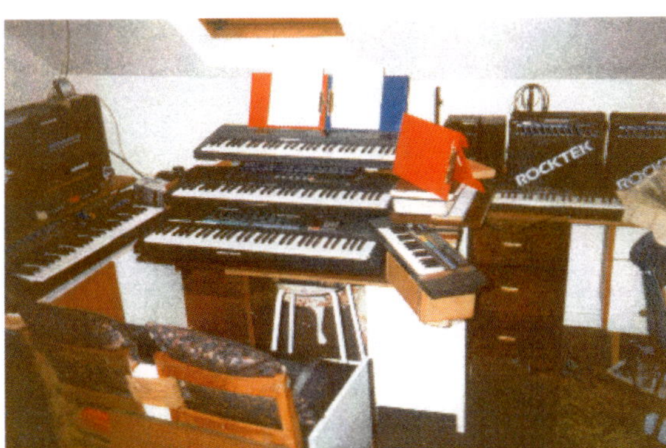

Dad's kingdom.

Then he inherited a stray dog called Scamp. My life was never boring and we did laugh so much as underneath it all me and my dad were on a similar wavelength a little bit bonkers. The bath and the rest of the flat harboured his obsession for collecting rubbish and he looked like the local tramp as he wandered the streets dishevelled and unkempt, but he was protected from harm by those fearful staring eyes that stared straight through you for most of the time – empty, lost eyes that held no memory of his past life. There were only glimmers of the man we once knew and they lasted only for a short time before paranoia took over. When we visited I became attuned to his change in mood and would make a quick exit when this happened. We didn't have the power or the money to lift him out of this world of deprivation and I loved the times I didn't visit to avoid the fact I was helpless in the ability to help him. Money is not everything but it does speak volumes if you have it.

Within the community Dad was exploited by prostitutes, people pretending to be his friend to rob him of his benefits. When he insisted on stopping his medication and threw a ghetto blaster at my car with the children in it, I had to stop visiting for a while and life was peaceful. There were some very guilty times when I wished his cruel life would end but I questioned honestly why! Who was I to judge? I know one thing: I didn't feel I was safe to visit again until they realised his vulnerability and he was moved into a residential home where he had freedom and also supervision and safety. I then began to visit again. When I was undergoing cancer treatment I didn't tell him I had cancer and he never asked about my new-fashioned hair attire, a scarf covering a very bald head. We visited as a family and my brother Adrian would play the keyboard and sing 'Let It Be' by the Beatles. I would join in and we would all as a family sing happily together embracing our mutual love of music. In 2009 the family had visited Dad and we had on video a family rendition of 'Let It Be' with me singing and dancing in the background, happy, glad to be alive spending these precious times with my dad, brother and sister – Adrian playing keyboard, Helen filming – and by now we had Erica my granddaughter standing at the side of the keyboard just beginning to get the taste for the family love of music.

Two weeks later my brother was dead. He had kept to himself the fact his own mind was starting to enter the turmoil he knew his own father had suffered at the very same age, thirty-nine. The situation was further complicated by the end of his relationship and his isolation and loneliness just prompted him to take the option of suicide.

IF ONLY

Why didn't he call me and say
Help me, help me I plan to die?
Did you think of me,
Think of Mum,
Think of Helen?
We all would have run to you,
Picked you up and carried you for a while
Until you felt well enough to walk the path of life again,
To face the world and smile.

Looking In: A Hospital in Birmingham, UK, June 2011

I am standing at the top of the ward looking down at all the patients' faces. I can see some are recovering well and chatting to their relatives, some are asleep. They might as well be as it saves them from the pain of knowing they have nobody visiting them tonight. Then some are lying in bed so ill they do not know it's visiting time. I stand here and feel I have been transported back in time standing here in my navy-blue dress and frilly white cap in charge of the ward, a newly qualified staff nurse looking down the ward at my patients. It is visiting time and now I am responsible for not just the patients but for the health and safety of the relatives.

I remember the famous ward round at visiting time and we would ruffle the visitors' feathers when we would firmly say, "Only two to a bed, please." Ten or more relatives would gather round the bed as if it was the patient's front living room, desperate in their own way to show that they were there to see them because they loved them, but forgetting the risk of bringing in infections from the outside world that may compromise the one they love's recovery.

I notice an older lady with a walking stick, head bowed, sadness in her face as she talks to the man lying in the bed. The elderly man is fragile in appearance. I see in this older lady's face recognition that life as she knew it so many years ago, that brief moment captured, will soon become a distant memory. I see the nursing sister looking over and walking towards this lady to comfort her and I quickly join her to listen to what she has to say. I see myself thirty years earlier in the same role on this very same hospital ward comforting relatives – such déjà vu. I hold the older lady's hand because the man lying in the bed is my father – I hold my mother's hands.

Weeks later Mum was in Wales, which was good. Mum had said her goodbye that very night we had visited the hospital. Helen and I were called to the nursing home, in fact the whole family turned up, a reflection on our family philosophy of family loyalty. We sang 'Wish Me Luck As You Wave Me Goodbye' and Dad squeezed my hand. He waited for me and Helen to leave, before he took his last breath.

DAD

The disease of the mind is hard to define
An island separated
By an ocean in turmoil
That stops your mind
Meeting mine.
In the early days we swam in a calm clear blue sea,
My sister, my brother, and me.
We would swim to the shore and rest on the softest sand
A family together united hand in hand
But one cold and thunderous volatile grey day
The ocean became angry and swept the family away.
A wild and destructive wave came sweeping over me
A family all drowning in sadness
And unpredictability.
In your final years and your final days
The sea became calm and we swam through the waves
To rest on the shore on the soft, soft sand
At last we could reach you, united again we stand.
I turn to my sister as a bright light begins to shine.
I say to her,
"I have waited.
It has taken a lifetime
But I just captured a moment,
A moment so sublime.
It was that precious moment when
At last
My Dad's mind
Meets mine.

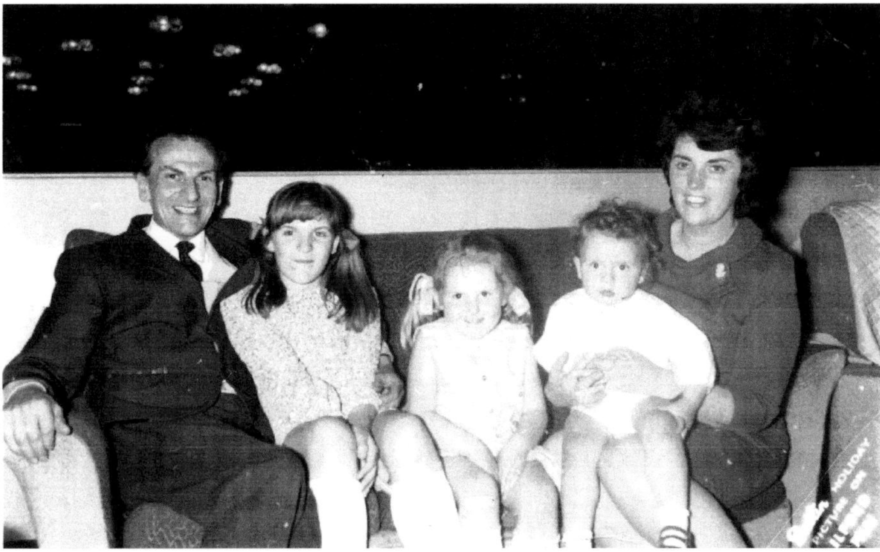

Before the thunder. Butlins holiday, 1970.

Looking In, 11 November 2011

Five months later, a maternity ward in Birmingham, UK.

Here I am again five years later on labour ward for the second time this week with Fiona, my daughter, who is being prepared for a caesarean section. I should not be here not about to share a miracle of life with my daughter, not again. I look at the small-framed fragile girl, yes my baby girl in the bed, she has been sick all the way through her pregnancy and she looks more like my baby girl than a woman awaiting the birth of her own child. I am smiling in anticipation and joining in with the excitement of the miracle that is about to happen but there is a part of me that feels like an imposter, a gatecrasher at a party, a party that should be private between

Fiona and the father of the child but for reasons I could never understand he chooses not to be here. I am her mum and she needs me and I am here, full stop. And I am fuming.

WHAT EVER HAPPENED TO DADDY?

My daughter telephones Baby Father
He is pondering about his day;
In a hospital nearby
You tell him
A miracle is about to happen,
His baby boy is on his way.

Why aren't you here?
I think to myself
To see my girl crying
He's watching TV
Apparently I'm told
A chat show his cue;
In a hospital nearby
I am watching over your son
Where are you?

Why aren't you here?
To see my girl crying

Baby Father has promised to visit
To see his own flesh and blood
We wait patiently my girl and I
Did you come?
No
If only you would.

Why aren't you here?
To see my girl crying

Baby Father sits in his castle
Alone for many years to come;
In a nearby town
We live
A happy family,
Never lonely in life.
We have the love of your
Growing son.

We don't need you
Here
We are all SMILING.

Looking Back

I walk the length of the labour ward to get myself a drink and as if transported by a time machine I trace my steps as a young student midwife walking briskly up and down a ward filled with an air of nervous tension mixed with excitement and that is just the midwife. I remembered working and being paid for a job that on a daily basis allowed me to share life's miracle. I would be privileged to share this special moment in a lifetime. I would have tears in my eyes. The responsibility factor of a midwife for these two precious lives is totally daunting and for not one minute can your concentration or professionalism lapse. The expertise of the midwife should never be underestimated.

As I look at my sleeping daughter, I see a familiar face and that face is me twenty-two years ago not walking the floorboards as a midwife, no, a picture of me in labour. My husband, who was standing next to me, was merely an onlooker, there in body but not soul. The labour became more fraught and my life hung in the balance. I felt the softness of a hand holding mine, a calming reassuring voice whispered in my ear. It was not my husband but the Doctor telling me that if my heart rate continued to rise any further, I would be rushed in for a caesarean section. Childbirth is not always a fairy-story miracle and I had also been a part of tense times and emergencies and sometimes tears had been not those of happiness but genuine tears of tragedy.

After five painful miscarriages, this baby was precious, I had nearly lost him at twenty-six weeks pregnant. Now my son was in danger of losing his mum!

I came home with my beautiful baby boy. Soon the hard reality was that my own family was to soon fall apart. Just four months after the birth of Ali, my husband and I separated.

It was time to find another career path that took me away from the repeated reminder I had failed in my marriage. Single-parent world with a weekend dad. Ali was four months old, Fiona was five years old, and so I left my married life with two children and about five black plastic bags. I went to live with my sister-in-law and her husband. I was even more upset to have to leave my extended family whom I had grown to love over the years.

A few months later I found the perfect job in a GP practice as a treatment room sister. I loved my job as a practice nurse, and with my fresh enthusiasm for my new role I earned the title of practice nurse finalist 1992 – 1992 was a good year for me and I married again after a wedding preparation of two weeks to my second husband. I was happy again in a stable relationship with the family life I constantly yearned for and a new baby. I was fulfilled and happy again – well, for now.

Wanting to further my career I started university again and commenced my health visiting training. I would take my assignments to bed after the children were all settled in their beds sleeping. It was hard work combining parenting and university but there is always a happy ending and I started working part-time as a health visitor in 1994. Health visiting was a culture shock, now working in the community on the front line my role was to support families, prevent ill health and provide the generic population with advice and education about how to stay healthy and keep out of hospital. I must have loved my job because I stayed for fifteen years in the same job in the same town working with the same wonderful people who are my forever friends as well as colleagues. I did move onwards and upwards at one stage in my career. I had an opportunity to be Assistant Locality Manager, with responsibility for three community hospitals and the NHS Trust community workforce. Little me in a big, big job. I could have continued in this role but for two reasons: my dicky ticker started playing up, and Lisa my youngest daughter had the opportunity of touring the country with a ballet company, BRB. I needed to give her my commitment and time, and at the same time still work to pay the bills and also attend to the different needs of all three children. I had to make a choice again: work or family. Neither really won the day it was more the fact of choices always being influenced by one main issue, health. I had to look after myself, but I had to reduce two stresses, the home/work balance and financial stress. We moved to a smaller house – well, you will laugh at this story – we moved back to the road we had moved from six years ago. All I can say is I am glad I didn't fall out with the neighbours. It was fate because we didn't choose to go back but we did a house swap with the couple who purchased our present house. I returned to part-time working. Stress levels decreased only to be replaced not long after our move by the stress of cracks appearing in my marriage.

Sure enough after Lisa left to start her education in Tring in Hertfordshire we moved into a rented flat in the town, a luxury flat and local to Ali's secondary school. I again took on a promotion as Health Visitor Service Manager. My management Bible was *Feel the fear and do it anyway* by Susan Jeffers. Fiona was working in The Mailbox in Birmingham. I had in the last few months gained strength and made a decision that my second marriage had reached the end. Although there was the fallout of such a major life event to contend with, for me and the children life became peaceful. I was blooming with health and happiness. I had reached a point in my life when I couldn't have been more fulfilled. My children were well, thriving, doing well in education. Lisa was fulfilling her dream as a dancer. I had reached the point in my career when I felt proud of myself and so very proud to be managing a community nursing service I believed in.

Happy memories that's a fact.

Health Visitor Explained

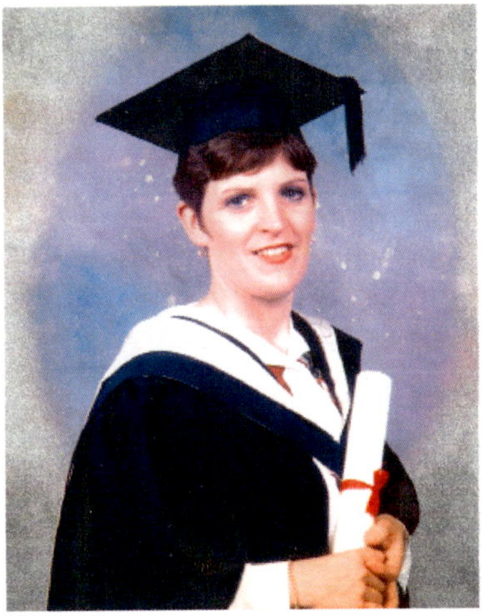

Retail is not my ball game as I found when I started my little printing business selling bookmarks and notepads. I am hopeless and I give everything away and profit is a word I used rarely in my entrepreneurial days as a business lady. I have learnt to stick to what I know best although with a small contradiction to this statement. There is a moral to the story, I did know best when I was selling my health visitor community nursing service when a Health Visitor Service Manager. I believed so strongly in my profession and the benefits of having health visitors in the community nursing team and the invaluable contribution to the NHS health visiting is not quantitative it is qualitative and very hard to measure in a cost exercise. With this in mind I just relate to you the simplest scenario. To give you an insight to what I am talking about.

A mum comes to the baby clinic with her baby, I see her entering through the door and immediately I read her facial expression and as others pass her by I see she is hesitating at the door and turns to look behind her as if to walk away. I walk over and smile at her and welcome her into the busy clinic setting. She doesn't smile back but sits down head bowed and waits her turn The baby is eight months old and starts to cry. It's loud in the baby clinic and she is frightened. I turn to look over to see what is happening and I see a baby distressed and looking searchingly at the mum's face but there is no recognition in her eyes. She reaches into her bag and mechanically gives the baby a dummy, the baby stops crying a while when she realises Mum is not listening and there are two sad expressions now looking around. I walk over and call the baby's name. We weigh the baby and talk about feeds and Mum answers me in monosyllables, head bowed and with no eye contact. The baby has lost weight but Mum is insistent baby is feeding well and her hands begin to shake. It is time for me to ask that question – the one health visitors know so well – and I had checked there was a private room and warned my colleague I might have to leave her single-handed to run the clinic for a while because I had already made my assessment and possible reasons for Mum coming to clinic today. So I go ahead and asked, "HOW ARE YOU?" I rest a hand on her shoulder to let her know I am there to listen to her and make time for her and as I thought she begins to cry and tears trickle slowly down her cheeks. I hand her the tissues and lead her to a room where we can talk in private and there we start a programme of support for herself and her baby's emotional health. A happy mum does make a happy healthy baby.

And the moral of the story is that the baby clinic is not a morning out weighing babies; it is a collective opportunity to monitor the health of mum and baby in a holistic approach. We may see twenty to thirty or more babies and parents in one morning and each contact can bring with it the routine intervention of checking a baby's weight. There may also be a need for active intervention, more serious issues such as postnatal depression, child protection, housing and benefit issues, relationship problems including disclosure of domestic violence. The public health arena is actively ongoing in the clinic setting with visual displays designed by the health visiting nursery nurse team; posters and prompts to better family health care i.e. healthy eating, smoking cessation, signposting to other voluntary agencies, e.g. Home-Start, Women's Aid and more. Finally the clinic is then filled with a few tears as babies and children are cuddled by parents after receiving a childhood immunisation to protect them and their tiny peers and community from infectious diseases.

So that is what happens at the health visitor baby clinics. Any questions, anybody? This same scenario I quoted at a meeting with GPs, who wished to cut the HV service – that didn't happen! By the way the government decided to train more of us.

I would say I was for this moment in time the happiest I had ever been in my adult life. I had my career I loved so much, a reasonable income, healthy happy children all of them achieving. My passion for salsa dancing and the wonderful community of salsa friends that came with the dancing. I was my healthiest and fittest and happiest.

In September 2005 I returned from my first fun girlie holiday in Magaluf and I found a lump in my breast and so my first book was born, *Single Salsa Survivor*. I was diagnosed with breast cancer on 30 November 2005 and life changed. As in my third book, *Always Sublime, Never Ridiculous*, life became sublime but never ridiculous. I was a different person leading a very different life but I was still very, very happy.

Not long after my treatment I received an insurance policy and some money to spend and I was intent on treating my friend Salsa Jill to a salsa weekend in the sun.

Nursing does not stop when you leave your shift. You live and breathe the responsibility of the NMC code of conduct and this can run into your private life whether you like it or not. If you can help within your professional scope of practice then you should help whether on the streets in a shop or even 35,000 feet in the air.

Once a Nurse Always a Nurse!

Salsa dancing is my addiction in life and my salsa dancing took me to Santa Susana, Spain. I had seen the weekend advertised and felt very proud of myself as I booked a self-made holiday in Santa Susana ready to join all the other salsa community in Barcelona. Wow, I was so excited and I was going with my fellow salsa best friend, Jill. Two days before we were meant to fly Jill jumped up in the air at a netball game and wham, ruptured Achilles, no salsa dancing for Jill, and so Lisa was told to get her passport and get her case packed.

We turned up at the airport to find a few other salsa dancers heading for Santa Susana and the salsa weekend celebrations – well, so we thought. The first hilarity happened right there in the airport. Our new-found salsa friend led us all on to a train to our destination and we followed only to find we were going in the wrong direction. She made the sound of a sheep as we had all followed a local on to the train and we laughed and laughed and laughed and the weekend bond with our friend had formed. We then boarded the train back in the right direction. We stood there taking in the scenery and coastline of Costa Blanca, suddenly a Madonna song filled the carriage and a human-sized puppet danced along the carriage. How surreal that was! I just hung on to my euros and my daughter, bemused but exhilarated by the random start to a random holiday.

We reached our destination and walked along the promenade looking for our hotel. The others had found their hotel and we were left just me and Lisa walking looking for the hotel. We found it and we were pleased it was a lovely hotel. I did notice one thing: we were the only salsa weekenders in the hotel. Uhmmm. The salsa weekend in Barcelona was a formal organised weekend away and although I felt a little daft and stupid we just joined in. I would have never imagined I would ever be a gatecrasher, how embarrassing. Fortunately I knew many of the salsa dancers and they embraced Lisa and I into the salsa fold. Lisa and I would sunbathe in the day and enjoy our mother/daughter quality time. It was just a good job Lisa can dance because we would dance all night. There was no excess alcohol consumption, everyone was totally focused on the dance moves as usual and a perfect twizzle meant no unsteadiness caused by alcohol. I met two other salsa addicts who were also single like myself as Lisa quoted a saying from *Bridget Jones's Diary*. We all then became Bridget and to this day I cannot remember their names.

To the airport with happy memories but the surprises were not over yet and the next thing I knew there was mayhem in the cabin. The commotion made us aware there was something not quite right and an aura of panic was creeping down the cabin.

A voice shakily shouted, “Is there a doctor on board?”

No answer.

A rather more urgent voice shakily asked, “Is there anyone with medical knowledge on the aeroplane?”

Lisa looked at me as if to say, “OMG no, Mum, why always you?”

I looked around the cabin for any other offers of help but there were just anxious faces looking at the person sitting beside them for inspiration.

I heard my own voice say, “I am a nurse,” but didn’t have time to say I was recovering from cancer treatment and feeling just that little bit lacking in confidence. I didn’t have time for self-sympathy and so the NMC code of conduct just ran through my mind and it was all systems go. It would have been negligent of me not to try and do something to help this person. I knew I might have to make an instant life-saving decision. The next thing I knew I was witnessing my new-found salsa friend struggling to breathe. A first-aid kit with a bandage and nasal spray was available. I quickly made some decisions and shouted for Lisa to bring my purse. I had in my purse aspirin that I take before flights because tamoxifen has an increased risk of thrombosis. I had Piriton in case I had another allergic reaction like that I had experienced after my cancer treatment had finished.

I managed to ask my friend a few questions. She

had the feeling her throat was swelling and her chest was tightening, she was breathless, her pulse was rapid. But she could at this moment still swallow. I made an instant decision to use what I had got. I had no choice, her airways might be cut off by the time we landed. I encouraged her quickly to take the aspirin. I was lucky she could confirm she didn't have asthma as a rule or any allergies that she knew of. But this was either a heart condition, a pulmonary embolism or a severe allergic reaction and so I gave her Piriton as well. Another thing they had on board was oxygen, and I administered that and the nasal spray, intent on doing anything to keep those airways open. I took out aeroplane seats and lay my friend in the recovery position and I sat on the floor by her face monitoring colour and pulse as she settled and relaxed caused by the effects of the Piriton. The pilot asked if we should land in Paris or not and I had to make a decision. Her condition had settled, so I said carry on to Birmingham – it was literally twenty minutes away, but notify the ambulance service to be ready to board the plane and take her to hospital.

I landed with no seat belt and I thought I was penned in anyway and I was not prepared to leave my patient. We landed and everyone except myself and Lisa got off the plane. The ambulance was on its way and the pilot came through the cabin in all his splendour and thanked me for what I had done. I was, underneath it all, frightened that I might not have made the right decision and I hoped I had not caused her any harm, and then I reassured myself that I had coped well and as the paramedics put drips in and on a trolley transported her from the plane to an ambulance I left escorted through the airport, flip-flops and all. Lisa was not phased that much because life was never boring when with her mum; there was always something going on if Mum was about.

I thought a lot about my salsa friend and what had happened to her and a few months later at a big salsa dancing event I heard a scream above the music and a familiar face came running towards me and hugged me and thanked me from the bottom of her heart for saving her life.

We hadn't known names as we had called each other Bridget the whole holiday and she could not trace me to thank me.

I was eternally grateful to her for still being alive and confirming that I had made the right medical decisions.

Thank God for that.

Looking In, 28 February 2012

It is never a bad thing to reflect on your past and one very valuable lesson is to learn something positive about yourself or even something you might not even like about yourself, sometimes, but you are you and if we are open to change and consider life a learning curve then we will never have regrets.

Author Susan Jeffers considered herself a recovering know-it-all and said, "I don't really know everything but neither does anybody else."

Sting from The Police, a group from the early 80s, was asked what he disliked in life and he said, "Blind certainty, because underneath is a desire to be right and this causes tension." The MAYBE world eases this tension. I believed maybe I would survive cancer maybe I wouldn't, but for now I would live my life to the full. I have no regrets in my life but I might have done things a little differently maybe even as recently as my relationship with my husband as in my last book, *Living in Grief, Loving in Grief: The Story of Loss and Love*. In Hindsight, if we had a crystal ball, led by instinct when I met my husband who had lost his wife to cancer I tried to heal a broken heart and also help his grieving daughter. The nurse instinct was in action. We do have to recognise our limitations and for a while I thought I could nurture and help, but I am not a nurse in this situation. The only person who can help her is her dad and her loving sister.

In 2012 as I brought Donell, my grandson, aged five months through my door to live with his sister, Erica, and for me to parent him as I had Erica five years ago, so Chris, my husband, walked out on 6

May, not to be seen as my husband again – it was over!

I returned to work as a school nurse in January 2012, and I struggled from May to November juggling parenting and working. I retired again! My manager and friend said she would not buy me another retirement present. We laughed and I retired with my promise to use my writing skills to shout from the highest mountain how valuable the School Nursing Service was to the schools, the children, the parents, the teachers and the community.

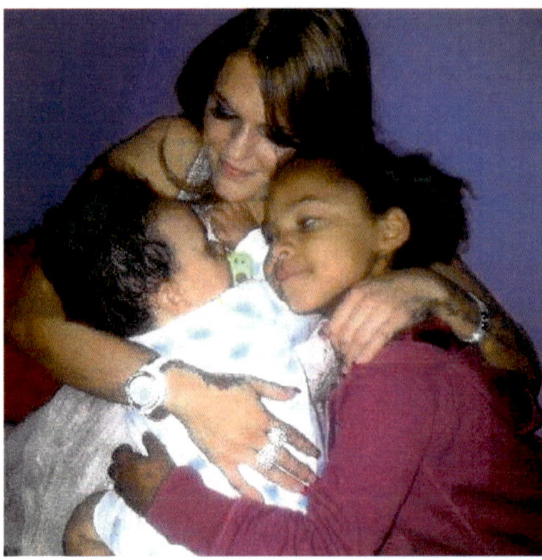

Donell moved in.

Sharon Rose's Message

Today the sky is the limit
The future is as secret and deep as the ocean
Tomorrow is a blank canvas
The promise of life's masterpiece
A dream for now
There is no magic potion.

Capture the excitement
As your life before you
Mysteriously unfolds
Paint your world
With bright colours of the rainbow.
Take a chance
You have a choice
Positive thoughts
Will lead you to your
Very own pot of gold.

Good luck
And goodbye for now.

So I have looked in, looked back, looking forward is now a fact. My long-term goal is of course to still to stay alive sharing that goal with my sister of course and I leave you with a Sharon Rose message.

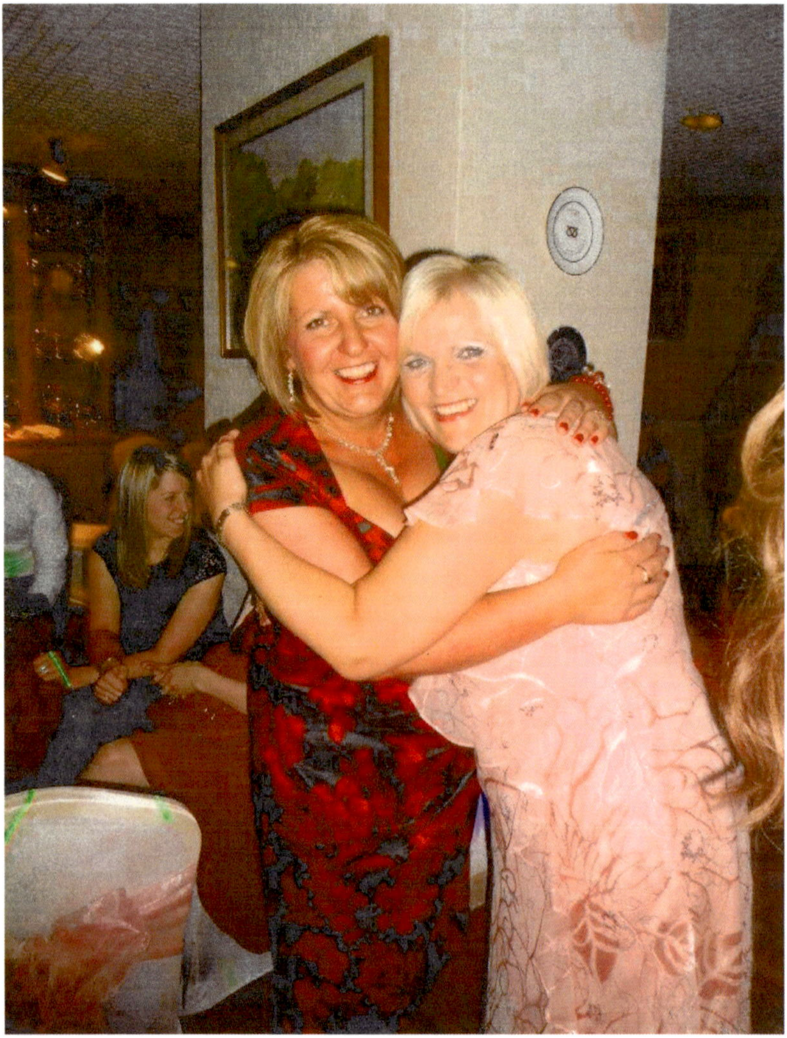

The author and Helen at Ali and Leanne's wedding, 2012.

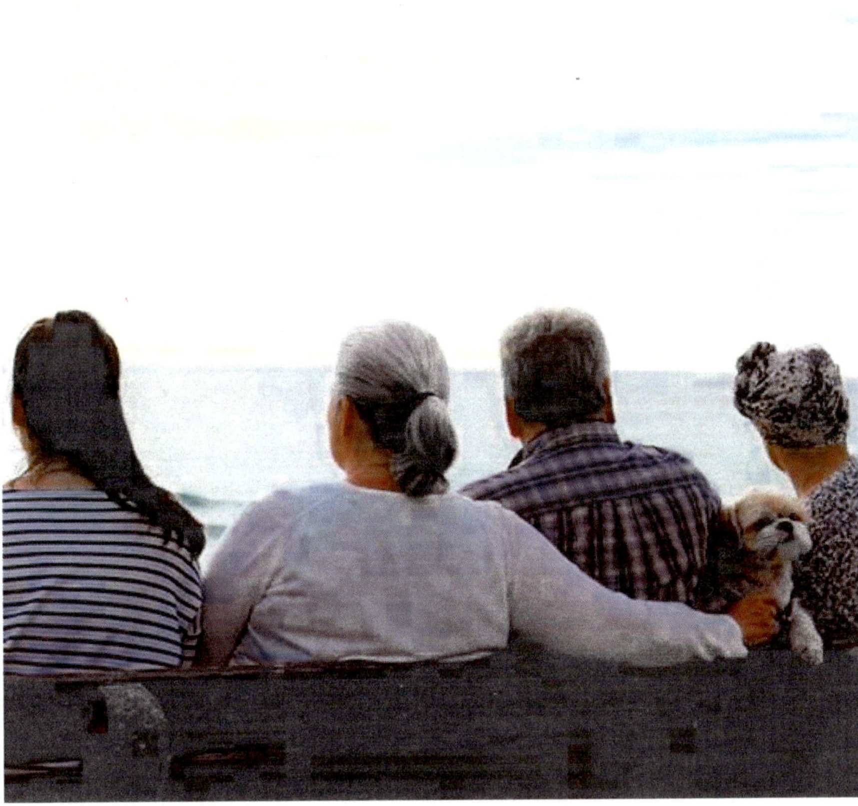

Never look back, only look forward ~ by Sarah Jones

This is a recent photograph taken in Cornwall in 2015. My dearest, wonderful friend and Health Visitor colleague who is presently 'Looking In' as her daughter is being treated for Hodgkin's Lymphoma. Their strength as a family.

Daughter-in-law, Leanne and grandson, Louie outside the church after Louie's Christening .

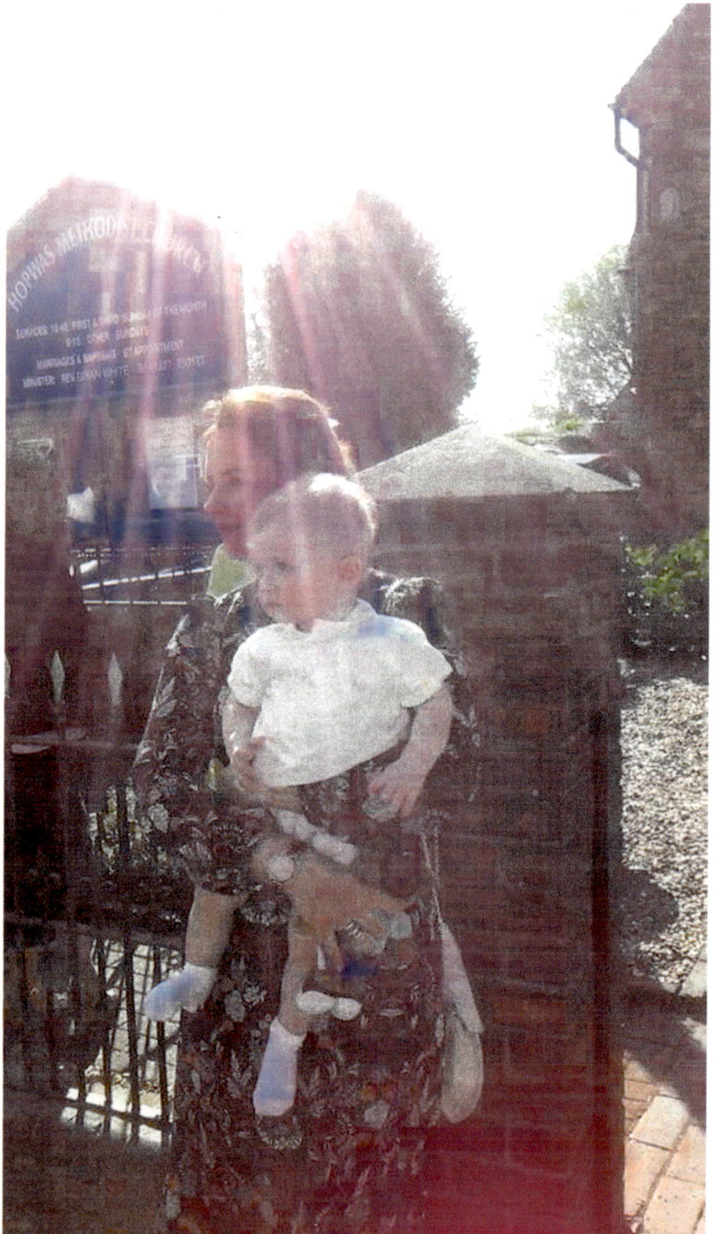